Edgar Cayce Cures

Using Alternative Holistic Remedies and Treatments

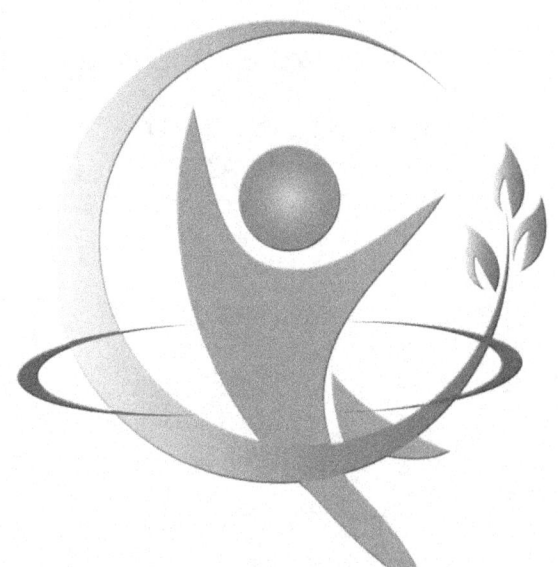

B. A. Anderson

Copyright © 2012 - B.A. Anderson

Edgar Cayce Cures
Using Alternative Holistic Remedies and Treatments

All rights reserved. No part of this book shall be reproduced or transmitted in any form or by any means, electronic, mechanical, magnetic, and photographic including photocopying, recording or by any information storage and retrieval system, without prior written permission of the publisher.

EdgarCayceCures.com

LOC: 2012948487
ISBN (978-1479248483) Paperback

Published by DM BookPro
Phoenix, AZ
DMBookPro.com

Available Now on Amazon
Edgar Cayce Cures - All My Lives Journal
(Using Akashic Records to Heal)
Edgar Cayce Cures - All My Lives Workbook
Edgar Cayce Cures - All My Lives Workshop CDs

Coming soon:
Edgar Cayce Cures - Diabetes and Blood Sugar Levels
Edgar Cayce Cures – Using Ideals and Spiritual Principles
Edgar Cayce Cures - Journal to Heal
Edgar Cayce Cures - Using Akashic Records

Dedication

This work and all of my work is dedicated to Spirit for all their Love, Guidance and Protection and for that I am ever grateful!

Thank you

Contents

Introduction	6
Recommended Herbs	10
Body – Mind – Spirit	11
Atomidine	15
Castor Oil	19
Charcoal Capsules	27
Charred Oak Keg	33
Formula 636	35
Glyco Thymoline	39
Ipsab	43
Limewater	47
Mullein Leaves	49
Radiac	51
Violet Ray	55
Wet Cell Battery	59
Bonus Material	
Poultices	63
Case Studies	73
Index	79

Introduction

What sort of person turned to Edgar Cayce for medical information?

What did it mean for someone suffering to receive advice from the Father of Holistic Medicine and America's most famous clairvoyant?

The A.R.E. library in Virginia Beach contains 14,246 copies of Edgar Cayce's psychic readings, steno graphically recorded over a period of 43 years. Of this number 8,976 or 64%, describe physical disabilities of several thousand persons with a suggested treatment.

Cayce looks at the human being as a three-dimensional manifestation of a spiritual reality. He states that man as we know him is composed of energy which is in a state of homeostasis, a physical body that we can see and feel.

Principal Concepts of the Cayce Approach to Health and Healing

The Cayce approach to health and healing is based on the following fundamental concepts:

- **Holism** - This approach affirms that human beings are multidimensional including physical, mental and spiritual aspects which must be considered in relation to health and healing.

- **Inner Healing** - All healing comes from within. Our bodies have the inherent ability to be healthy. Therapeutic interventions work best by assisting the processes of innate healing.

- **Prevention** - Healthy lifestyle is emphasized as a means of staying well and preventing disease. Because all healing comes from within, the same therapies which assist the body in healing itself are often helpful in the prevention of illness.

- **Self Care** - Self responsibility in making choices and applying what we know to be true on a regular basis is the foundation of health. Many of the therapies utilized in this approach are best done in the home and as part of the daily routine of life. The Cayce Herbal contains a special section that addresses the use of simple herbal remedies in the home for common ailments.

- **Natural Therapeutics** - "Nature cures" is the basis for many healing systems as it is for this one. Natural remedies and therapies which work closely with and are supportive of the body's innate healing ability are emphasized in this approach. Therefore it is no surprise that herbal medicines play a significant role in Cayce's approach to health and healing.

- **Integration** - The Cayce approach acknowledges that all therapeutic modalities and systems of healing can be helpful. The important point is to find the best combination of treatments for each individual. This cooperative attitude seeks the common ground between systems and is known by various names such as "complementary medicine," "integrative medicine," and "comprehensive medicine". - "The Cayce Herbal" contains numerous practical examples of this principle, especially with regard to integrating herbal therapy with diet and nutrition, manual therapy, electrotherapy, and hydrotherapy.

- **Individuality** - Each person is a special entity. Health and healing can best be achieved by a person-centered approach that recognizes and utilizes the uniqueness of each individual rather than limiting people to diagnostic categories and pathological labels. Although the disease-centered (allopathic) model is utilized in certain sections of The Cayce Herbal", it must be recognized that a more individualized approach is ultimately more effective and is certainly more consistent with Cayce's philosophy. The challenge of individualized assessment and treatment planning must also be acknowledged.

- **Health & Illness** - Health is a state of wholeness, balance and growth. Incompleteness and imbalance ("incoordination") are common experiences which can challenge us to grow and develop. Thus illness can often be viewed as an opportunity for transformation.

- **Non-Invasive Assessment & Treatment** - "First do no harm" should be practiced with regard to assessment and treatment. Practitioners should seek the least invasive procedures available that can assist with inner healing. Keep in mind, however, that surgery and/or medications can be helpful for extreme situations. Since herbal medicine tends to be milder and less invasive than standard medical treatment, the role of botanicals in the Cayce model is emphasized.

- **Cause and Effect** - Although symptomatic relief to decrease suffering is desirable, addressing the underlying cause(s) is also strongly emphasized in the Cayce readings. One of the strengths of the Cayce approach is the wealth of insight into the patterns of "cause" and "effect" associated with the various categories of disease.

The Cayce Herbal contains numerous insights from the Cayce readings on fundamental etiological and pathophysiological processes which can be therapeutically influenced by herbal medicines, particularly when integrated with other natural modalities.

Edgar Cayce recommended herbs

Aconite	Ipecac	Juniper	Potato
Agar	Camphor	Lavender	Prickly Ash
Aloe	Canadian Balsam	Lemon Juice	Psyllium
Alum Root	Capsicum	Licorice	Pumpkin Seed
Anise	Cascara	Lobelia	Ragweed
Arnica	Castor Oil	Mandrake	(Ambrosia)
Arrowroot	Catnip	Milkweed	Rhubarb
Asafoetida	Celery	Mullein	Sage (Clary)
Balm of Gilead	Cinnamon	Mustard	Sage (Garden)
Balsam of Peru	Clover	Myrrh	Sarsaparilla
Belladonna	Cloves	Olive Oil	Sassafras
Benzoin	Cocoa Butter	Onion	Senna
Black Haw	Coffee	Opium Poppy	Slippery Elm
Black Root	Cola	Passion Flower	Snake Root
Black Snake Root	Dogwood	Peanut Oil	Squill
Blackberry Root	Elder Flower	Peppermint	Stillingia
Blood Root	Eucalyptus	Peruvian Bark	Strychnine
Buchu	Fennel	Willow Charcoal	Sugar Beet
Burdock	Fig	Wintergreen	Tobacco
Calamus	Foxglove	Witch Hazel	Tolu
Calisaya	Friendly Fever	Yellow Dock	Turpentine
Camomile	Ginger (Wild)	Yellow Root	Valerian
Grapes	Ginseng	Yellow Saffron	Verbena
(Concord)	Golden Seal	Plantain	White Pine Oil
Horehound	Jimson	Poke	Wild Cherry Bark
Indian Turnip			

Body Mind Spirit

Spirit is the life - Mind is the builder - the Physical is the result!

Edgar Cayce was perhaps the most famous and most documented psychic of our time. He is known as the Sleeping Prophet and the Father of Holistic Medicine.

For more than 40 years, Edgar would lie down on a couch and go into a light sleep state and responded to questions. These sessions called readings were carefully transcribed by his secretary and preserved by the Edgar Cayce foundation in Virginia Beach. Nearly 9,000 of the readings are health related of the over 14,000 recorded readings.

As the Cayce readings suggest: to better understand our bodies we must view ourselves as being composed of three parts- a physical body, a mental body, and a spiritual body. Each is separate from the other and at the same time they are one and the same thing. Each of the bodies can be worked on within its own realm and yet they are constantly affecting each other. Change in one is reflected as a change in all of them.

Life is a journey with a purpose and with a destiny that we must come to know ourselves and yet be one with God our source.

Cayce spoke of man or woman as an eternal being originating in the spiritual realm and having an ultimate destiny back to the spiritual realm. In the interim, we pass through many incarnations here on the Earth plane.

Cayce spoke about each of us as body, mind and spirit in unity; the spirit of God is the life, the mind is the true builder, and the body is the result of what the mind has done with that power we call the spirit. True healing is always marked by an awakening process within the cells, the atoms, and in the tissues of our entire being.

A number of mind-body techniques were recommended in the readings to individuals in their attempts to get well:

1. Visualization exercises
2. Breathing techniques
3. Working with dreams
4. The role of positive emotions
5. Meditation
6. Affirmations

These techniques should always be used in combination with the suggested remedies or treatments for a complete body-mind-spirit healing.

The cells within our body have the ability to renew and regenerate themselves; this is the most fundamental of all universal laws. The human body can rally its healing forces and repair itself with more vigor than the world's best trained medical team. The Cayce readings are clear that this healing ability and ultimately all healing is a direct result of the manifestation of spirit within our body.

Looking at the physical body, the Cayce readings described the physical points of contact for our spiritual bodies as our glands which secrete that which enables the body physically to reproduce itself.

The seven endocrine glands are special vortexes of energy that correspond to the chakras.

To understand the healing process we must see ourselves as a body-mind-spirit entity. There is a oneness that encompasses all three. There is an energy that connects all three—the life force. We should look at ourselves as an ongoing stream of consciousness; a creation that is constantly changing even as we think about it; a being shaped by our experiences—both constructive and destructive—in this life and in many past lives.

Drs. William A. McGarey and Gladys McGarey started the A.R.E. Clinic in Phoenix, Arizona, in 1970. There were many healings accomplished at the clinic for patients who found little relief from conventional medicine. This was attributed not only to Drs. William and Gladys McGarey and the unconventional remedies found in the Edgar Cayce readings but also his philosophy of healing the body mind and spirit.

The Clinic treated and healed its patients for more than 40 years. But, after the death of Dr. William McGarey, the clinic struggled. During the Clinic's last year in 2009, while I was helping with some marketing efforts, Edgar Cayce came to me psychically and told me that I would be part of the changes happening to the clinic very soon. Within a week, I became the last director of the 40 plus year old clinic during its final months. I promised to continue the education of the Edgar Cayce principles and Drs. William and Gladys McGarey's dream.

This book contains the most talked about remedies and the ailments that the Edgar Cayce readings mentioned and those used in treatment at The Edgar Cayce Clinic.

The pictures displaying the product brand are given to you in this collection because there are only two manufactures' that follow the Edgar Cayce recommended ingredients. Those two companies would be Heritage and Baar, they both produce and sell the products from their online stores but these recommended products can be purchased in many places online or in some local natural or health food stores.

We hope that this book can be used as a quick reference handbook to keep with you, to easily reference the Edgar Cayce remedies and therapies.

Barb Anderson

Atomidine

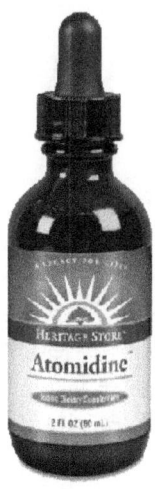

Atomidine is "atomic iodine," less toxic to our bodies as compared to the iodine found in kelp tablets. Atomidine is a unique iodine preparation that Cayce said would be extremely beneficial for many health purposes.

Approximately 610 of Cayce's readings suggest **Atomidine** in cases involving a glandular deficiency or a shortage of iodine in the system. According to Cayce, it may be used wherever there is an indication of an unbalancing of a gland, and may also be used as preventative.

Atomidine was rarely prescribed as a treatment by itself but was used as part of various programs.

Atomidine was recommended at The Edgar Cayce Clinic routinely and can be used for many ailments (refer to index to see all the possibilities besides what is stated in this chapter).

This versatile solution naturally supports:

- Energy
- Weight Loss
- Metabolism
- Calcium absorption
- Glandular function

Iodine is an essential nutrient to the thyroid gland and the entire glandular system. The thyroid is responsible for the production of hormones which regulate the metabolic rate of cells. Therefore, it influences physical and mental growth, nervous and muscle tissue function, cardiovascular health as well as healthy weight maintenance.

One of three factors that make calcium available to the bone is iodine. Atomidine is a wonderful supply of iodine, easy to handle, absorb, and eliminate.

Though Atomidine is a safe external remedy for anyone, it should be used internally with care and with a prescription.

Ingredients: 600 micrograms of iodine per drop (400% RDI).

Directions: 1 drop in water in the morning.

Warning: To avoid over-stimulation of the thyroid gland and resulting nervousness, do not use this supplement in conjunction with any other concentrated source of iodine, such as Formula 636/637, Sea-Adine, Calcios, or kelp tablets (not kelp salt). People who are hyperactive or have cardiovascular difficulties should not use this because glandular stimulation might overexcite the heart

Testimonials

Atomidine

"I used Atomidine under the direction of a doctor for Hodgkin's Disease and it worked excellently."

From Kansas

Atomidine was used for fever sores in my mouth and within three days it was healed. It usually takes two weeks for them to heal."

From Arizona

Atomidine provides the stimulation necessary without the side effects of that thyroid medicine that the doctors prescribe.

A woman in New Mexico

"I seem to more energy and have less depression since taking Atomidine. My health is improved.

From California

Before using Atomidine, tests showed very low thyroid. I took the Atomidine as directed, under an osteopath's guidance, and numerous tests since then have shown normal thyroid function. It is a tremendous product. Also, I think it is fantastic for sore throats.

Woman from Texas

"I was taking the Atomidine for mouth ulcers and noticed an immediate improvement. I was cured in three days. This is the only product that has ever given relief."

A Pennsylvania woman

"Atomidine works quite well to provide immediate relief from sore throats."

A New York woman

"Atomidine is excellent. I used it for an ingrown toenail and it corrected the nail and also eliminated the infection."

A South Dakota woman

Castor Oil

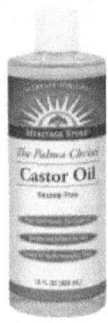

Another name for castor oil is Palma Christi, or the palm of Christ. It is appropriate that a plant used for so many healing qualities to be named after Christ.

Castor oil has a variety of external uses such as mixing castor oil and baking soda for calluses on the feet, moles, ingrown toenails, and warts.

Castor Oil Packs

Castor Oil packs were advised in about 570 readings and most often used for:

- Inflammation of the gall bladder
- Poor eliminations
- Epilepsy
- Liver conditions
- Headaches
- Appendicitis
- Arthritis
- Colitis

Then in an additional 50 readings castor oil was recommended for:

- Massage
- Cysts
- Bunions
- Moles
- Tumors
- Warts

It seems as though Castor oil is good for everything that ails us. The amazing thing is that nobody really understands why Castor oil is so effective. More amazing is that most modern doctors don't use it, either because they don't believe it works well or because they think it's old-fashioned. If all medicines that we use were as effective, we would hardly have any sickness.

How to use the castor oil pack:

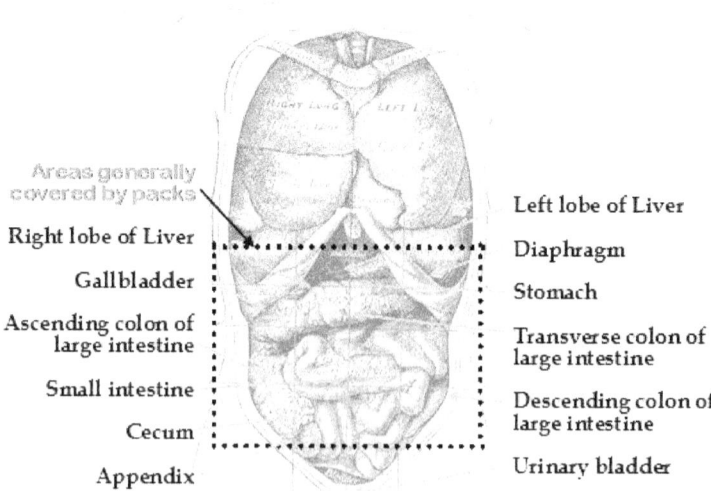

Instructions:

Take a piece of soft flannel cloth or wool flannel if cotton flannel is not available, fold three or four times, and end with a pack that is approximately 8 to 10 inches wide and 10 to 12 inches long. This is the size needed for the abdominal application. Other areas may need a different size pack. For some castor oil onto the cloth make sure the cloth is wet but not dripping with oil. Then apply the cloth to the area that needs treatment.

Apply a plastic covering such as Saran wrap over the soaked flannel cloth. On top of that place a heating pad and turn it to low to begin, adjusting the temperature as the body tolerates it. Then wrap a towel folded lengthwise, around the entire area and fasten it with safety pins. The heating pad should remain in place between 1 and 1 1/2 hours only. The pack itself can be worn all night. Be extremely careful to avoid excessive heat.

The skin can be cleaned afterward by using soda water (add 2 teaspoons baking soda to a quart of water).

The flannel pack can be kept in a plastic container for future use. It is possible to use the same pack for different problems, and it need not be discarded after one application.

Other conditions that castor oil has been used for are allergies, animal bites and stings, arthritis, calcium deposits, cancer pain, cuts and abrasions, cysts and tumors, hair and nail problems, epilepsy, eye irritation, flu, hair growth, injuries to the head, legs, ankles, back, fingers; knee pain, lesions, nausea, palpitations, moles, warts, punctures, getting cancer, snoring, sprains, and wound healing.

True stories:

I was giving a **Cayce** remedy workshop demonstrating some of the remedies and treatments from the **Edgar Cayce Clinic** formally known as the **ARE Clinic**. We were talking about the use of castor oil and the Violet Ray appliance. A mother and her two daughters who were present for the lecture began to talk about one of the daughters (let's call her Betty) having a recluse spider bite. The spider bite had gotten quite large with a gaping hole looking red and inflamed. The other daughter (let's call her Nancy) decided to use the **Edgar Cayce** treatment of castor oil and UV Ray appliance. So Nancy applied castor oil to Betty's leg where the spider bite was, then placed plastic wrap over the castor oil pack and let it sit for about an hour. After removing the plastic wrap and oil pack, the wound appeared less red and somewhat better. Nancy then used the **Violet Ray** appliance touching the glass ball directly on Betty's wound and passed it around the reddened area for about 10 minutes. The open wound appeared to have gotten smaller. Nancy then reapplied the castor oil pack and sent Betty to bed for the night. Upon waking the next morning, Betty felt that the bite was less painful. Nancy removed the **castor oil pack**, cleaned up the oil on Betty's leg, and found that the wound was less than 1/2 the size it was the day before and it was barely red it all.

Nancy then applied the **Violet Ray** appliance as she did the day before for about 10 min. Again, the wound appeared to be growing smaller as she used the appliance. She continued this treatment of alternating castor oil and **Violet Ray** appliance treatments throughout the day. When Betty got up on the third day, the wound was practically gone, completely closed with just a little pinkness around the edges.

Another lady I knew told me she was experiencing great stomach discomfort or pain in the upper abdomen. I told her about the **castor oil treatment** and she decided to try it. She applied the castor oil pack over her stomach area, placed the plastic wrap over that, and used the heating pad for about an hour. She removed the heating pad, felt somewhat better, but left the oil pack on for the rest of the evening. She awoke in the morning with no stomach pain, her lower back felt better, and her only complaint was how messy the castor oil was.

There was a woman who was told that she had a fibroid tumor in her uterus. She started using the **castor oil packs** by soaking the cloth, placing it over her abdomen, putting on the heating pad, and lying there reading. As soon as she got sleepy she removed or shut off the heating pad and went to sleep, A couple hours later, when she decided she needed to turn, sure he moved the heating pad and the oil castor oil pan, and went back to sleep. She had continued this for about six months. At her six-month checkup, her doctor told her that the fibroid had disappeared.

Why does this work?

It appears that with various conditions the packs have the effect of stimulating the activity of the lymphatic streams while at the same time enhancing the elimination of toxic substances from the cells locally where the castor oil is applied.

When an area that has been injured, or isn't flamed, for one reason or another, is treated with the pack, the cellular tissue is capable of responding more normally with toxins removed. So they can take care of the infection or inflammation.

Another example of castor oil treatment occurred after a man smashed his hand between two rocks. There were no fractures, but the hand was badly scraped and bruised. A warm castor oil pack was applied to the hands. The next morning the results were dramatic. The swelling had completely subsided and healing had occurred at an incredible rate. By the third day, the healing was complete. The remarkable thing (other than the healing) was the absence of pain after an hour following the application of the oil pack.

History:

Cayce gave thousands of medical readings while in a trance. During these readings, **Cayce** recommended the use of castor oil packs 575 times for menstrual cramps, lymphatic disorders, and other medical conditions.

Dr. William McGarey wrote a book titled *The Oil that Heals: A Physician's Success of* **Castor Oil Treatments**, where he further gives case studies using castor oil.

My main reason for writing this book is to help others know that the **Edgar Cayce Clinic** (formally the ARE Clinic) in Phoenix used and proved the healing qualities of Cayce's readings by treating patients successfully for over 40 years.

Testimonials

Castor Oil

"An X-ray was taken of a woman's breast, small tumors the size of peas were seen. A couple larger ones were drained with needles. She was told that when they become larger they would she would need surgery. She started using Castor Oil packs on her breasts at night. She went back for X-rays the following year and the tumors were gone" –

An Alabama woman

"Several years ago I was having a terrible pain in my wrist and it made a clicking noise when I moved it. When the pain became worse and constant, I finally went to my doctor. After x-rays, he found a cyst that was strangely formed and made an appointment for me to see a bone specialist. A week later I saw the specialist who again x-rayed and determined that the cyst was congenital, thus accounting for the strange way in which it had formed. The cyst had nothing to do with the pain that was tendonitis. He recommended cortisone shots when I could tell exactly where the pain was. My whole wrist hurt. I give you all this background just to point out that no treatment was given – nothing even suggested lessening the pain – and it cost more than $120.00! My sister suggested Castor Oil that I purchased for 79 cents and applied the treatment a couple times a day for two or three days. The pain and the clicking noise were one and have never returned!"

a woman from New Mexico

Fibromyalgia and Castor Oil Packs

After being diagnosed with fibromyalgia for many years, and my symptoms became increasingly worse. Tylenol seemed like my best friend, I was able to make it through the day

I had read about the use of castor oil packs and was more than willing to try anything to relieve the pain I was having.

I thought using a castor oil pack seemed like such an old-fashioned treatment. I have a new lease on life, after a few days I noticed there were no more body aches, I didn't need to take Tylenol anymore. I was sleeping better and I have more energy, I am so full of life and grateful for my new life.

It's like magic, it works; and such a relief for me.

JS from Arizona

Charcoal Capsules

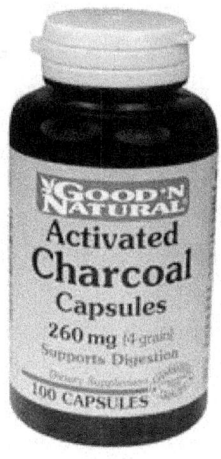

Activated Charcoal

Charcoal tablets were prescribed in about 15 readings for digestive problems and flatulence.

- Aides in digestion
- Great for abdominal bloating
- Gas discomfort

Activated charcoal (a.k.a. active carbon, adsorbent charcoal, and medicinal charcoal) is a fine black carbon powder made from natural materials such as wood pulp. Due to its large surface area, activated charcoal has high adsorption properties; it keeps certain substances from being absorbed into the stomach.

The Cayce readings advise, only take them when necessary to keep down those tendencies for gas formations. Activated charcoal is an insoluble black fiber traditionally used to absorb a variety of substances.

Using activated charcoal:

Dosages will vary depending on the reason for supplementation. For those desiring reduction of LDL cholesterol levels, recommended dosage is 500 to 1000mg as needed. Activated charcoal is available in the following forms: capsules, enteric coated tablets, granules, liquid, and tablets.

Side effects and cautions:

This may cause black stools, diarrhea, nausea or vomiting in large doses. Do not use activated charcoal if you are without anatomically intact gastrointestinal tract, or have any bowel obstruction. Activated charcoal should only be taken 2 hours before or 2 hours after consumption of food, nutritional supplements or medications.

Charcoal is harmless and there are no known allergies to it.

Activated charcoal can be used for some of these situations:

Bad Breath

Add 1 tablespoon to a glass of water. Stir it well and drink freely. Then add 1 tsp in a half glass of water; rinse your mouth out with it. Be sure to swish it around in your mouth for a few seconds before spitting it out.

Mix a small amount of charcoal with water to make a thick paste. Brush your teeth and tongue with it. Your toothbrush will turn black; but no worries, you can easily rinse out the charcoal. A definite bonus is that brushing with charcoal can help to whiten your teeth.

If your breath is really bad, drink several glasses of charcoal water during the day and rinse out your mouth with charcoal water after each meal.

If you have ongoing problems with bad breath you may have an infection in your mouth, or there may be a problem somewhere in your digestive system. Visit your dentist and doctor to rule out any other health conditions that may cause bad breath.

If your bad breath is caused by indigestion, use a *charcoal poultice (see poultices) over your liver and abdomen. To avoid indigestion, it is very important for you to practice healthy eating habits.

Bee Stings

Charcoal can help soothe the pain from a bee sting. Mix some charcoal powder with enough water to make a paste. Smear the paste on the bee sting. If you've got a lot of bee stings, fill your bathtub with warm water. Add 2 cups of charcoal and soak in it. Follow that with a charcoal compress.

Diarrhea

Take two heaping teaspoons of powdered charcoal 4 times a day as well as with each loose stool. Cut the dose in half for a child. Be sure to consume a lot of clear liquids such as vegetable broth, herbal tea (red raspberry, chamomile, and peppermint are good choices), and diluted juice to replace electrolytes and to prevent dehydration. See your doctor if you don't see any changes in your condition.

Food Poisoning

Charcoal is very effective for food poisoning. Take 1 tablespoon of charcoal in a glass of water. Then drink another glass of water. Do this each time you have a loose stool.

Foul Odors

Get a jar with a lid that has holes in it. Fill it with powdered charcoal. Place the jar in a place where it will not tip over. You can place the jar in your closets, the fridge, your drawers, or anywhere that is prone to bad odors.

Gas (Flatulence)

If you find yourself passing a lot of gas, try charcoal (see below for dosages). It will absorb the gas very quickly and give relief.

Indigestion

Take 1 to 2 heaping tablespoonfuls stirred in a little water. Indigestion can cause bad breath. Follow the directions above for bad breath.

Nausea and Vomiting

Charcoal is effective for nausea and vomiting. Stir 1 to 2 tablespoons of charcoal into a glass of water. Follow with another full glass of water. Cut the dose in half for a child. Every time you vomit, you should take another full dose, even if you have to keep on repeating it.

You can make activated charcoal into a poultice or compress to help with many different conditions including abdominal pain, arthritis, bug bites, earaches, sore throats, sprains, and more.

CHARRED OAK KEG

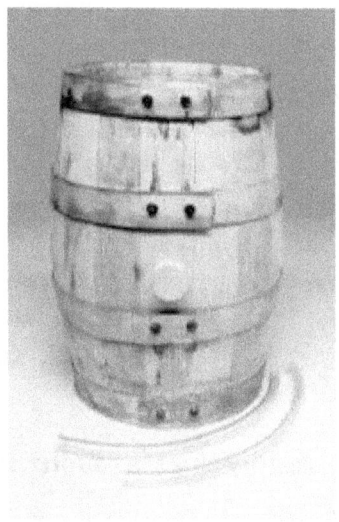

Recommended for the Throat and Lungs

Introduction:

The **Charred Oak Keg** is an American folk remedy for the lungs and has been used at the **Edgar Cayce Clinic** (A.R.E. Clinic) for decades. It appears to be helpful in resolving virtually any kind of abnormal condition in the lungs. Its effectiveness probably stems from a stimulation of the circulation of blood and lymphatic fluids, and by this mechanism it would relieve bronchial spasms, clear the lungs of toxins and lesions, enhance immunity to bacteria and viruses, and improve a diminished respiratory capacity.

Illnesses that seem to be positively affected by this simple traditional remedy include:

- Emphysema
- Scleroderma
- Lung cancer
- Valley fever
- Tuberculosis
- And many others

While you do not need a doctor's approval to begin using this remedy, for best results you should contact a doctor familiar with the **Charred Oak Keg** so that your therapy can be coordinated properly.

For more mild respiratory illnesses such as:

- Asthma
- Bronchitis

The **Edgar Cayce Clinic** (The A.R.E. Clinic) used the Inspirol inhalant, which is used in the same manner as the **Charred Oak Keg**.

Instructions for Use

Remove plug from the side of the keg. Place the keg in a bathtub or other large container and completely immerse it in water for 48 hours. This soaking will cause the wooden slats to swell and the seams to seal. Remove it from the water, drain it, and let it dry overnight.

With the keg on its side, fill the keg halfway with two bottles (fifths) of either 80 or 100 proof apple brandy. When not in use, keep the keg tightly corked and in a relatively warm area - but, of course, away from conditions that might ignite the alcohol. The warmth usually results in a greater concentration of apple brandy vapor in the keg, and this makes the treatments more effective.

To take a treatment, insert a plastic tube (1/4" to 1/2" diameter, usually provided) into the keg, keeping the inserted end above the level of the liquid. Place the other end of the tube in your mouth - like a straw - and inhale the brandy fumes slowly and deeply into your lungs. If you find this makes you cough, you must inhale more slowly.

Hold the fumes (if you can) for a count of 3, and on future occasions try to extend the count to 10 or even 20. The treatment works better the longer the fumes are held in the lungs. Also, the length of time you can hold the fumes is an indicator of the degree to which you have improved. A person with no respiratory problems can inhale the brandy vapor deeply with no problem and can hold it for as long as they can normally hold their breath.

Frequency of treatment:

Take a total of four inhalations from the keg. That is considered to be one treatment. The minimum number of treatments a person can take and still see improvement appears to be four treatments a day, each treatment separated by several hours. For a more severe illness, it is better to use the keg more often, taking treatments as often as once every hour.

When the fumes become weaker, the keg can be "recharged." It normally takes about six months for the brandy to lose its strength, but improper corking can reduce this time.

To recharge the keg you must empty it and re-soak it as given above and then refill it with new brandy. If you fail to re-soak the keg, you will probably find that in a month or two your keg will begin leaking. If you notice that your keg is leaking, pour the brandy from it into a container, re-soak the keg, and put the brandy back in. If the keg still leaks, it is time to get a new keg.

Most conditions are resolved before there is a need to buy a new keg.

People using the **Charred Oak Keg** will often benefit from using the **Inspirol** remedy as well, as the keg cannot be transported in a vehicle (it counts as an open container of alcohol); and it cannot be used in most work environments. **Inspirol**, however, can be taken with a person wherever they go, and it doesn't leave an odor of brandy upon the breath.

The **charred oak keg** was recommended in the **Cayce** readings about 50 times primarily in cases of tuberculosis and pleurisy. In fact, **Cayce** cured his wife, Gertrude, of tuberculosis at a time when TB was often a death sentence. The doctors thought that such treatments were useless, however, two days later Gertrude's fever diminished. Several months later she had completely recovered from tuberculosis.

Formula 636

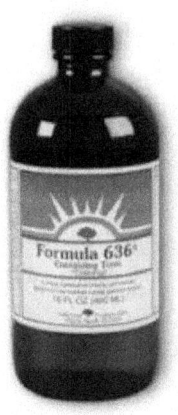

Formula 636

Cayce's energizing formula for men and women will help.

Naturally increase energy. The formula is an unusual combination of herbs and other substances high in essential vitamins and minerals.

Recommended for:

- Restoring natural color to gray hair
- Energizing
- Nails
- Complexion
- Support healthy hair growth and youthful color

Formula 636's unique blend contains:

- Atomidine with iodine to support normal metabolism glandular function, weight loss, and energy
- Ginseng (100 mg) helps counteract sluggishness and gives you an energy boost
- Phytoestrogen Black Cohosh (100 mg black snake root) has been documented in many studies for its role in balancing dramatic hormonal shifts and alleviating PMS and menopausal symptoms. Contains liver extract.

Other Ingredients:

- Iodine (250 mcg)
- Vitamin B-6
- Elixir of lactated pepsin (400 mg)
- Liver extract (200 mg)
- Black snake root extract (100 mg)
- Essence of ginseng root (100 mg)
- Also contains water, sugar, and alcohol

Directions: 1/2 teaspoon after each meal for 10-day periods alternating with 5-day rest periods. Other possible dosage: 3/4 teaspoon after morning and evening meals only.

Caution: If you are pregnant or nursing, seek the advice of a healthcare professional before using. Do not exceed recommended dosage unless instructed by a doctor. KEEP OUT OF REACH OF CHILDREN. Note: If this tonic is used in conjunction with any other concentrated source of iodine, such as Atomidine, kelp tablets (not kelp salt), or mineral supplements, over-stimulation of the thyroid gland with resulting nervousness may be experienced.

Testimonials for Formula 636

Formula 636

"With Formula 636 I feel better, stronger, no tiredness. It is a good way to overcome lethargy."

A Puerto Rico woman

My mother used 636 and she has arthritis. She can button her own clothes after she hardly finished the first bottle. She considers this miraculous, and she is no longer constipated. She is so delighted that she is telling all her friends.

A Virginia woman

"I thought I would mention that since using Formula 636, I lost 20 pounds, and don't have cravings for food like I did before. This has surely helped.

Man from New York

GLYCO-THYMOLINE

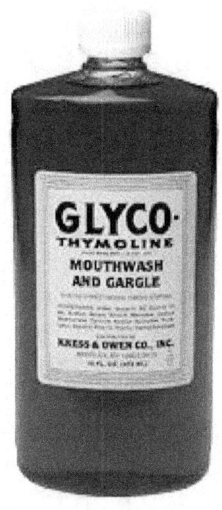

Glyco-Thymoline

- Mouthwash & gargle
- Alkalzing mouthwash
- Freshens breath

GlycoThymoline is an alkaline cleansing solution primarily used as a mouthwash and gargle. **GlycoThymoline** is used as part of an oral hygiene program or also for personal hygiene as it gives a refreshing clean feeling and is gentle enough to use on baby's skin.

Glyco-Thymoline is an original, unique natural formula. Originally, the exact formulation from the **Edgar Cayce Health Care Philosophy** and was referred to approximately 810 times in the readings.

Suggested Uses:

Oral Hygiene:

Use as a spray, rinse or gargle, diluted or full strength, as often as needed.

Teeth:

Use 1 part Glyco-Thymoline with 2 parts water (or full strength if desired) for cleansing between teeth with swishing action.

Baby's Skin:

Apply a solution, equal parts of Glyco-Thymoline and water to a baby's buttocks and genitals after each bath or diaper change, which helps to keep the baby comfortable.

Personal Hygiene:

Use equal parts Glyco-Thymoline and water to cleanse -genital external areas. Apply with soft cloth.

Intestinal Antiseptic:

According to the readings, when the system is overly acidic, cold and congestion can easily develop. Glyco-Thymoline was sometimes recommended to restore the normal acid-alkaline balance.

Ingredients:

Water, glycerin, SD (specially denatured) Alcohol 37 (4%), sodium borate, sodium benzoate, sodium bicarbonate, carmine, sodium salicylate, eucalyptol, menthol, pine oil, thymol, methyl salicylate.

Glyco-Thymoline Testimonials

"I have used Glyco-Thymoline packs for sinus infections and it cures it every time without drugs."

From Texas

"My experience with Glyco-Thymoline is this: I have had gum and teeth problems of long standing and had several extractions prior to my use of Glyco-Thymoline. I was told by a highly recommended specialist that he would not guarantee he could save my teeth, but he would make an effort and it would be expensive.

So instead I started using Glyco-Thymoline for gum massage and rinsing after brushing, as well as for a gargle as I like its soothing effect on my throat. I am holding my own with the teeth that I have - Thanks to Glyco-Thymoline."

From Rhode Island

IPSAB

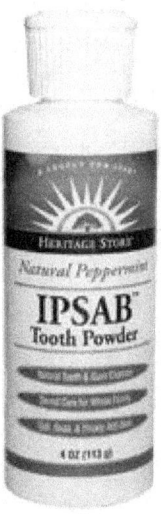

Ipsab Tooth Powder

In about 70 Cayce readings a solution of **Ipsab** was recommended for treatment of teeth and gums. A majority of the readings referred to a paste that might be made by adding salt in sufficient amounts to the **Ipsab** liquid.

This is an all natural salt and soda tooth powder with prickly ash bark and peppermint oil. The primary active ingredient is prickly ash bark traditionally used by Native Americans for maintaining healthy teeth and gums.

All natural Tooth and Gum Cleanser for the entire family, which has a refreshing Peppermint Flavor.

Suggested Use:

- Brush thoroughly with a soft bristle toothbrush and rinse with warm water.
- Massage the gums.
- Diluted form great for teething children.

Suggested therapeutic regimen:

1.-Treatment of early acute cases where gums are bleeding and teeth are loose.

- Massage gums for 5 minutes a day with **Ipsab** twice a day.
- Brush teeth once a day in evening with a mixture of table salt and sodium bicarbonate.
- Eat a large raw vegetable salad each day.
- Get any corrective dental done.

2. Prevention of pyorrhea, bleeding gums with no infection

- Massage gums for 5 minutes a day with **Ipsab** three times a week.
- Brush teeth twice a day and use salt and soda mixture at least once every other day.
- Eat a large raw vegetable salad each day.

Ipsab Testimonials

"My teeth and gums were in bad shape. After I used three bottles of **Ipsab** four times a week I had no infection and the trouble had cleared up. I consulted my dentist and he found no infection or disease."

From Louisiana

"I used **Ipsab** for the treatment of sore and bleeding gums. It has soothed and strengthened gums and stopped soreness. It also seems to reduce tartar formation."

A South Carolina woman

"I must tell you of the tremendous benefit that I received from **Ipsab** for gum treatment. My gums were red, swollen and bled with brushing or cleansing. Worse yet at times my mouth would fill with blood from the gums. The condition started to improve as soon as I started Ipsab and have steadily improved since.

A Pennsylvania woman

LIMEWATER

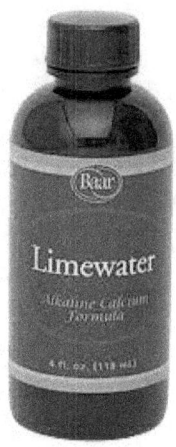

Limewater

Limewater is a saturated solution of slaked lime (calcium hydroxide) in water, used as an antacid. Limewater contains calcium and was often recommended in the readings for babies and children to aid in the development of strong bones and teeth.

Suggested:

- Indigestion
- Colic
- Pregnancy

Ingredients:

Calcium hydroxide, water.

Limewater Testimonials
Blood Cholesterol Down + More Energy

I have been using the limewater some time now and feel wonderful, having more energy.

I have checked my blood cholesterol and total cholesterol went down from 240 mg/dL to 200.

a man from Arizona

Arthritic Pain Gone!

I awoke this morning with my wrist aching from arthritis, about an hour after drinking the limewater the pain was gone, like magic! I will continue this wonderful cure

a woman from Nevada

Mullein Leaves

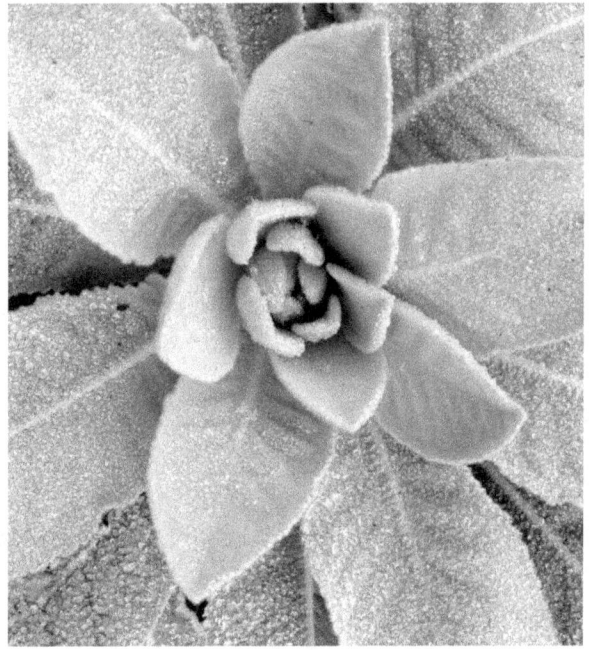

Mullein Leaves, 4 oz Herbal Tea

To ease the discomfort of:

- Varicose veins
- Supports vein health
- Supports healthy circulation
- Make a tea or poultice

Mullein tea was typically suggested by Edgar Cayce for supporting healthy circulation, especially through the urinary tract and lower limbs. From the Cayce health care philosophy:

Also, we would take internally a tea made from mullein. Pour about a pint of boiling water on the tender leaves of the Mullein and let steep. Make fresh each time. Do not try to keep over a 2 day period.

Suggested Use:

As a Tea:

Pour 2 cups of boiling water over a teaspoon of mullein leaves and allow it to steep as a tea for 15 to 20 minutes. Strain, serve and enjoy. Use 2 to 3 times per week.

As a Poultice:

Follow instructions for preparing tea. Allow to cool to body temperature. Strain and remove leaves and place on gauze or thin cotton cloth. Allow leaves and liquid to saturate the cloth. Place a heavier cloth on top and apply to desired area 1 to 3 times per week.

Radiac

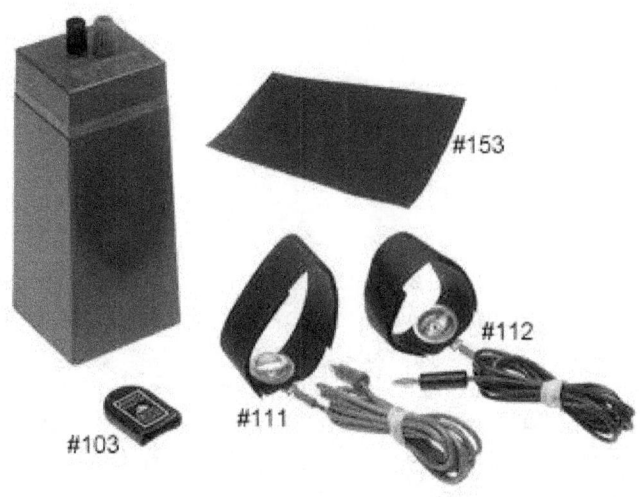

**The Radiac, with Extra Charcoal, Starter Kit®
Manufactured by Bruce Baar, MS, ND**

The **Radiac** has been called the meditation device, stress reducer, bio-electric balance and spiritual and self-unfoldment tool. Bruce Baar, the manufacturer of the **Radiac**, is featured in the books Super memory and SuperLearning 2000. The **Radiac** is also mentioned over 1,000 times in the Edgar Cayce Readings. (Pronounced: ray-dee-ack).

The readings recommend its use for the following:

- Particularly to improve circulation
- Normalize the functioning of the nervous system
- Aid in relaxing the body
- Reduce nervous tension

- Improve in coordination
- Lessen insomnia
- Diminish debilitation
- Minimize hypertension
- Reduce obesity
- Lessen arthritis

The appliance would be beneficial for almost anyone as long as directions were followed. In special cases a solution jar containing substances, such as gold chloride, silver nitrate, tincture of iron, spirits of camphor, tincture of iodine, or **Atomidine** for the purposes of vibratorally transmits certain needed elements from these solutions into the system. The effect of the solution in the circuit is to stimulate the system to produce the needed elements; the solution does not actually enter the body.

The appliance balances the vibratory rate in the bodily extremities. The **Radiac's** function serves to improve circulation and stabilize the nervous system.

There are about 200 readings recommending the use the **Radiac** at a time when the patient can be quiet and in a meditative state. It can even enhance your dream experience and even aid in spiritual awakening.

Some people call it the mind machine, the bio-battery, the radial appliance, the dry cell or the impedance device. No batteries and no electrical outlets are involved. To use it you place it in a plastic container, add ice up to the red line, then add water, wait 15 minutes and attach the leads (#111, #112) to opposite wrist and ankle as in the instructions. For instance, if you start with the right wrist, place the other lead on the left ankle. This forces coordination of the nerve reaction bilaterally. Relax and enjoy!

Designed for:
- Mental and spiritual unfoldment,
- Regeneration
- Attunement
- Memory enhancement

The **Radiac** balances the mental, physical and spiritual. Also enhances remote viewing and visualization while reducing stress. The **Radiac** is one of the best tools ever developed for personal growth. Be sure to order the Radiac book.

The **Radiac** is endorsed by the Association for Research and Enlightenment (A.R.E.), the Edgar Cayce Foundation, Health and Rejuvenation Center (H.R.C.), and the Cayce-Reilly School of Massotherapy.

The **Radiac** is to be used by only ONE PERSON. It cannot be shared. The **Radiac**, once used, becomes personalized.

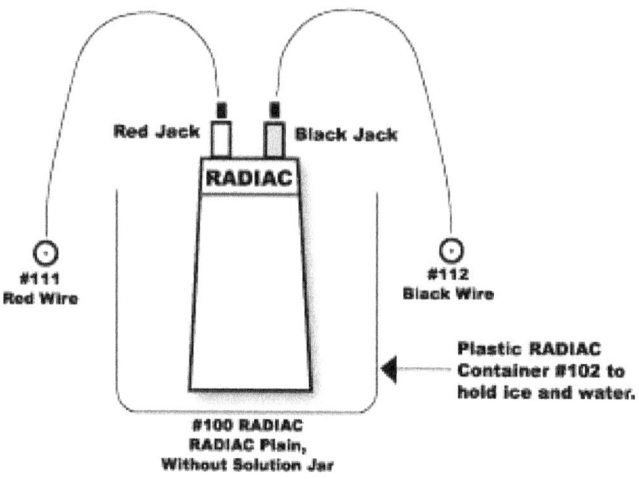

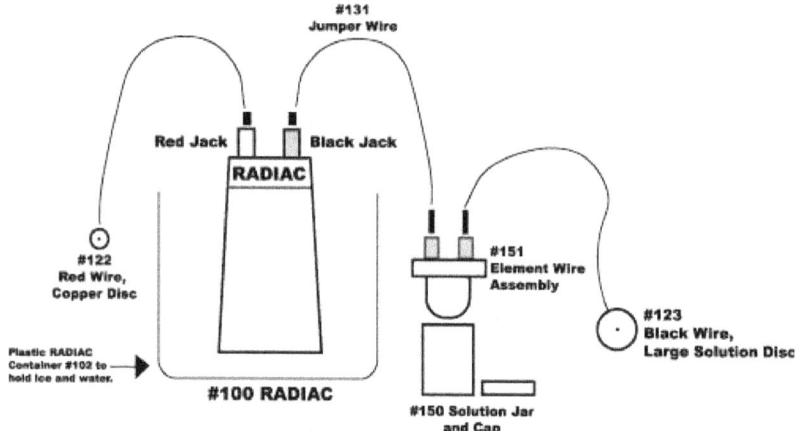

RADIAC® with Solution Jar Set

Violet Ray

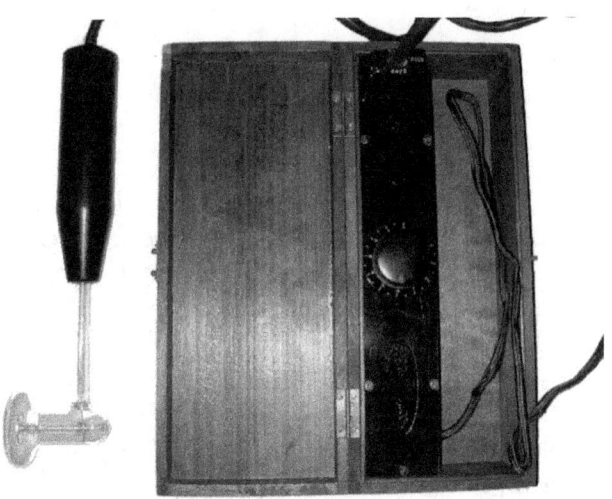

Violet Ray High Frequency Device
115v - for use in the USA

The **Violet Ray** or high frequency device is basically a low amperage source of static electricity and is detailed in the Violet Ray instructional manual.

Edgar Cayce refers to the **Violet Ray** in over 1000 readings given to individuals who sought his advice. **Cayce** believed the body, mind and soul are so closely interrelated, that it is rarely of value to treat any one of these aspects without also giving some attention to the state of the other two.

Recommended for:

- Circulatory system
- Hair care
- Menopause
- Nervous system

When the **Violet Ray** is applied, a surge of blood to oxygen-starved tissues stimulates lymphatic and capillary circulation, clearing cellular toxins and strengthening body organs.

The Violet Ray appliance is a handheld device with a variety of glass applicators. When the machine is turned on, a violet colored electrical charge can be seen. It emits warmth.

The **Violet Ray** is a **Tesla coil**, named for **Nicola Tesla**, the electrical engineer, scientist, inventor, and discoverer, who was granted 1,200 patents and is probably best known for his contribution of alternating current. Utilizing a transformer the voltage is increased dramatically as it moves through the resonation coil. The device's bulb contains a gas that ionizes and produces charged particles and that emanate from the surface. This combination of charged particles and high frequency produces a mild heating effect in the body. This heating of body tissue, called diathermy, increases the circulation, dilates superficial blood vessels, and promotes healing.

When recommended for someone with arthritis, it was said to relax the body, energize the nerves, and supply additional oxygen to cells and tissues.

It can be used with Carbondex®, carbon ash and Anidex®, (animated ash). Reference the Edgar Cayce health care philosophy.

It has an output of between 20,000 to 45,000 volts, at a frequency of approximately 500 kHz. The output of the Violet Ray is adjustable by means of a knob on the end of the unit.

Suggested Use:

This device is intended for intermittent use, no more than 10 minutes at a time. Never leave this device connected to the power line unattended. Remove from the power line when not in use. Use of a power strip with an ON/OFF Switch is recommended.

Wet Cell Battery

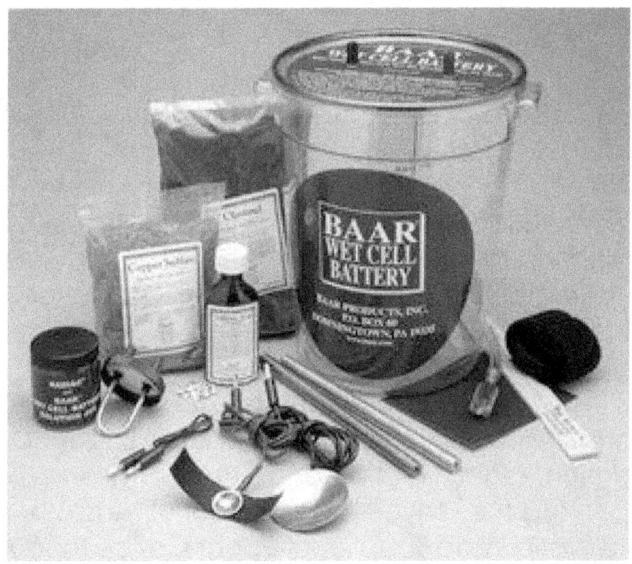

Wet Cell Battery

According to the Cayce Readings (referenced about 975 times) and The Edgar Cayce Clinic, this appliance is used for:

- A wide variety of physical and mental disturbances
- Incoordination of nervous systems
- Abnormal children
- Multiple sclerosis
- Insanity
- Arthritis
- Paralysis
- Parkinson's disease
- Deafness

- Rebuilding of tissue
- Restoring bodily functions

The **wet cell** is a battery, producing a very small electric current. This current stimulates the growth of nerve tissue, string fence the connections between nerve tissue. Specific solutions were to be included in the circuit, supplying certain elements to the body. The solutions most commonly used were spirits of camphor, gold chloride, silver nitrate, **atomidine**.

The Official **Wet Cell Battery** of **The Association For Research and Enlightenment (ARE**), **Edgar Cayce Foundation,** the Health and Rejuvenation Center (H.R.C.), and the Cayce-Reilly School of Massotherapy. Official World Wide Supplier of **Edgar Cayce** Products.

To begin using the Baar Wet Cell Battery:

You will need one **Wet Cell Battery** Starter Kit (pictured previous page).

For each additional month of use you will need:

- One Battery Charge Kit
- Two bottles of a vibrational solution

The Starter Kit is the way to begin researching the Baar Wet Cell Battery. It features a lightweight, non-breakable, clear container designed for visual inspection and ease of use.

Vibrational solutions such as gold, silver, camphor, etc., are purchased separately and will be determined by the information you are researching.

If more than one solution (gold, silver, etc.) is indicated, then purchase an Additional Solution Jar Set (#141) for each. The system must be replenished with new chemicals every 30 days.

Baar Battery Starter Kit Includes:

- #201 container with Lid - with instructions on lid for easy makeup
- #203 and 205 rods
- #122 small disc
- #123 large disc
- #131 jumper wire
- #142 extra wide Velcro belt
- #150 solution jar with storage cap (solutions sold separately)
- #151 loop with cap (element jar)
- #153 disc cleaning paper
- #215 one month battery charge kit (pre-measured battery components for 1 month)
- #133 brush with handle
- #217 mixing stick

Bonus Material Poultices

Potato Poultice

FOR EYE CONDITIONS

Background: The potato is closely related to the nightshades. Those parts of the potato that grow above ground and are exposed to light have the poisonous and narcotic properties of vegetables or fruit in the nightshades family. These portions are the stalks, berries and leaves. The fleshy portion of the potato that we eat does not contain these poisonous properties.

Only when young, green potatoes are exposed to light do they become bitter and poisonous. The tubers, which grow below ground, are enlarged portions of underground stems that become thickened in places where starch is stored. The tuber is composed mainly of starch and large quantities of potash salts. The raw juice from a mature potato contains a certain amount of citric and phosphoric acid.

Recommended for:

- Sty-bacterial infection of the eyelid
- Tired/inflamed eyes from overuse, contacts, crying and dust

Cleanses tissue/improves lymphatic drainage and draws out inflammation and infection of small eye irritations.

Edgar Cayce often recommended potato poultices (packs) for eye problems involving irritation or inflammation (such as blepharitis swollen eyelids).

Here are some specific recommendations for using potato poultices:

1. Use white ("Irish") potatoes or organic if possible
2. Use a potato that had been dug the previous year.
3. Wash potatoes thoroughly.
4. Use the peel and pulp by grating or scraping the potato
5. Use a piece of cheesecloth or gauze pads.
6. Close your eyes.
7. Place the gauze and grated potato over the affected eye(s) for 30 to 60 minutes each.
8. Wash the eyes with a weak solution such as 20% boric acid. For severe cases, the readings sometimes recommended washing the eyes before and after the potato poultice.

The frequency of treatment varied with the severity of the condition. Typically, the poultice was recommended to be used each morning and evening until inflammation and irritation subsided. The readings sometimes suggested cycles of treatment wherein the poultice is used for two or three days and then rest for a couple of days before resuming the cycle.

Onion Poultice
FOR EYE CONDITIONS:

Background: The common garden onion is one of the oldest and most versatile herbal remedies. Traditionally onion preparations have been especially effective in the treatment of colds and congestion.

Used externally, onion poultices have wide application including treatment of congestion, infectious disease, earaches, warts, athlete's foot, muscle pain, and unsightly liver spots or dark blemishes.

Taken internally, onion may be helpful for indigestion and circulatory diseases.

Recommended for:

- Respiratory System
- Colds
- Flu
- Chest Cough
- Bronchitis
- Pneumonia
- Congestion

It draws toxins, breaks up congestion and moves it through your system.

Prepare about six large onions, steamed in parchment paper. Squeeze out the juice and sweeten just a bit. Begin with small doses of the onion poultice taken about every two hours. This will change the condition of the stomach and the respiratory system.

Another method would be to take some onions and chop very fine or grind them. Mix with yellow corn meal about half and half and place on chest and throat and the lower portion of kidneys and lumbar area.

Grapes and Grape Poultice

GRAPE THERAPY

For abdominal discomfort associated with illnesses such as functional and inflammatory bowel disease, grape therapy was sometimes recommended by Edgar Cayce. Concord grapes were recommended be eaten, drank (as juice) and used in abdominal poultices. He insisted that the grapes contain the seed as the action of the tartaric acid in the seed are desirable.

The regimen for grape therapy varies depending upon the condition of the individual. Including quantities grapes and grape juice in the diet is encouraged.

A grape poultice should be used at least once each week. For acute conditions, and may be used almost continuously until relief is obtained.

Grape poultices key points are:

- Use crushed Concord variety grapes that have seeds, use the hull and pulp.

- Using gauze place about 1 to 1 1/2 inches of the grape hull and pulp between layers over the whole abdomen and leave in place until it is dry.

Grape poultices are suggested for lymphatic disturbances and the flu.

What Is a Charcoal Poultice?

A charcoal poultice - also known as a charcoal compress - uses activated charcoal to help lessen pain and pull toxins out of your body.

What Is Activated Charcoal?

Activated charcoal is carbon that has been treated with oxygen. This makes the charcoal more porous. Porous charcoal has more bonding sites, causing things to be chemically attracted to the charcoal. In turn, this allows the charcoal to trap the chemical impurities that cause infection, inflammation and other toxic reactions in the body.

Activated charcoal is used for a number of applications other than poultices, including in air purifying filters and water filters. It is used in fabrics and soaps, as well. It is also used as an odor absorber, such as in kitty litter and air neutralizers.

How Does a Poultice Work?

Poultices are believed to draw out substances from the body. In the case of a poultice made from activated charcoal, the porous properties of the charcoal attract toxins and then bond to them so that they leave the body and enter the charcoal.

Uses of a Charcoal Poultice

There are a number of uses for a charcoal poultice including:

- Pain reduction
- Pulling heavy metal toxicity from your body
- Reduce swelling
- Reduce inflammation
- Draw out infections
- Treat abscesses
- Treat bee stings
- Treat infection
- Minimize the pain and discoloration of bruising
- Heal burns
- Treat boils
- Minimize the pain and inflammation of bursitis
- Lessen the pain of earaches
- Treat inflammatory eye conditions
- Treat gangrene
- Draw out toxicity that causes liver disorders
- Provide pain relief
- Lessen muscle soreness
- Lessen the pain of sore throats
- Relieve itching from spider and bug bites
- Lower pain levels and treat swelling from strains
- Treat pain from tendinitis

These poultices can also be used to treat animals with similar conditions. Check with your vet before using a poultice made of activated charcoal for your pet.

How to Make and Apply a Charcoal Poultice?

To make a charcoal poultice, you will need the following items:

- Activated charcoal powder
- Water
- Some type of soft cloth such as gauze
- Plastic wrap
- Ace bandage or other strips of cloth
- Safety pins

Method:

Mix two to three tablespoons of activated charcoal powder with a small amount of water. Add just enough water to make a spreadable paste.

Spread the paste over a layer of gauze.

Cover the paste with another layer of gauze so that the charcoal and water mixture is between the two pieces of gauze. If you don't have gauze, you may also use a paper towel.

Place the poultice over the injured body part, taking care to make sure that gauze covers the entire affected area.

Place plastic wrap over the top of the poultice.

Wrap the entire thing with an Ace bandage or cloth strip and then secure it in place with safety pins.

Leave the poultice in place for up to ten hours, replacing as necessary when the poultice dries out.

Adding a few tablespoons of ground flaxseeds to the charcoal/water paste can help the poultice to retain moisture.

For small areas such as bug bites, sprinkle a small amount of water and activated charcoal onto the gauze portion of a bandage and place it over the bug bite.

Caveats and Cautions

If you are treating an area with mucous membranes, such as your eye, use a less porous cloth than gauze, such as a towel.

Never reuse a poultice - always make a fresh one.

Change out the poultice if the charcoal paste becomes dry.

Serious injuries, illness, inflammations and sprains need medical attention. Before you self-treat serious illness or injury, visit your personal health care provider for appropriate treatment.

Do not apply charcoal poultices to open wounds. If charcoal gets into an open wound, it will leave a permanent mark on your skin.

Case Studies and Testimonials

The stories that follow are outstanding examples of the dramatic ways in which healing has come to individuals via the **Edgar Cayce** readings. They illustrate that GOD does indeed work in mysterious ways. These case studies and testimonials were given after using **Edgar Cayce** principles, or using the **Edgar Cayce** remedies or receiving treatment from the **Edgar Cayce Clinic** in Arizona.

Case Study 1

My first Herpes outbreak occurred in August of 1976. To my satisfaction, and from visual observation, from the use Ray's ointment, **Slippery Elm Tea** and **Sulfax** I have experienced no more Herpes outbreaks. I used **Sulfax** for 5 days and I have continued daily with Ray's ointment and drinking one to two cups of Slippery Elm Tea, which I enjoy with orange blossom honey. **Ray's ointment** does stop the sting and itch.

Case Study 2

I am nearsighted to the point of needing glasses constantly. Late in 1977, I went to my eye doctor because I could hardly see out of my right eye. He diagnosed a pressure of 24 in my left eye and said 25 would require medication for glaucoma. He also found the beginning of a cataract in my right eye.

Three or four months later, I dreamt of an herbal formula, but couldn't remember anything but "balsam of tolu". I came into the Heritage Store a few days later and picked up a bottle of **optikade** and noticed that it had balsam of tolu in it. I went and read the Cayce reading on the product and decided to try it since it was a formula for the eyes. I used 8 bottles of the eye tonic over the next year. I also used castor oil packs, potato poultice over my eyes as well as steam baths and massages.

Late in 1978, I had another eye test and they found the eye pressure reading had dropped to 18, close to the level of 16. I also noticed the vision in my eye has improved substantially.

Case Study 3

I think it is important that I believed I was going to get well (Hodgkin's Disease) before I ever came to Virginia Beach or got involved with the readings. But prior even to the believing was a willingness to turn the whole thing over to GOD.

I had tried all I knew, doctors and very fine ones had tried all they knew, and there was simply nothing else to be done to say, Okay, God, you must know something I don't about this whole thing, and there must be something good about it that you'll let me know when you get ready to tell me or when I'm ready to hear or understand it.

I ran across the notion of and the procedure for meditation and it fit perfectly. You pray to God and then you listen to Him. I started it. Vey soon I experienced ineffable peace. It didn't matter whether or not I lived or died because God was my Father, just like, but very different from too, my earthly father. I'd always been in that relationship to God and always would be. It would transcend death and time and people and places and all that seemed right then to be very real and important.

I began to get well (my drug dosage, Leukeran, was reduced from three pills every morning to two and paradoxically getting well was no longer what mattered most. It was this new understanding about God and me that most consumed my attention. Later I moved to Virginia Beach on a temporary basis. I had planned to leave after several months to take up another commitment, but somehow that all got changed as I began to understand that following my intuition might be more important in some cases than living up to my word. At Virginia Beach, I was introduced to the readings on Hodgkin's Disease, met the Doctors McGarey and decided to go to their clinic the following summer 1971. I had already met a woman who had been cured of cancer at the clinic and I had made up my mind to be willing to do exactly what they suggested her to do. My conversations with her were the clincher on my commitment to go ahead and flow with it and see what happened. Certainly orthodox medicine had by that time failed to give satisfactory results with the Hodgkin's healing.

I spent two weeks in Phoenix, loved every minute of it. In addition to colonics and massage and the "normal Cayce diet" I took up drinking chaparral tea each day and inhaling apple brandy from a charred oak keg. How romantic! I was really getting into this healing business, having picked my own tea in Phoenix. I thoroughly enjoyed drinking the chaparral tea and sniffing the brandy, how much nicer than the death-like stillness and the ominous whir of cobalt machine. In addition to those therapies, Dr. McGarey recommended osteopathic adjustments, and castor oil packs applied to the abdomen, which I still do, and almonds, which I still eat.

By the time, I went to Phoenix, my hematologist at Duke University Medical Center in Durham, NC, had already stopped the Leukeran altogether. When I went back to him in the fall, I saw him in the hall, he said, "What's happened to you?, You look Great!" I had been seeing him since I was diagnosed with Hodgkin's in August of 1966.

Since June of 1971, there have been no active signs of it, and I know I am cured. I believe that Dr. McGarey was a channel for the healing I experienced.

Case Study 4

My child has been ill all summer long. It started with a simple cold, went into his ears, and the massive doses of oral antibiotics and shots threw him into a siege of diarrhea and vomiting that threatened to dehydrate him. After four rounds of oral antibiotics, two shots of penicillin, a round of Sulfa drug, and many concomitant decongestants to keep the mucus from pushing out from his nose to his ears and infecting them further I had spent almost $200, had visited our three pediatricians an average of twice a week for six weeks, and woke up one morning to my child's coughing and coming down with another cold.

I decided to check out **Cayce**, I ordered "Medicines for the New Age" and used it to make my decisions about what to order. I started giving cocoa butter massages, and added **campho-derm** massages, plus started letting him inhale from the **Inspirol** and take a one/third adult dose of the **636 formula**. You would not him as the same child after two weeks from the beginning of my cocoa butter rubs and the Inspirol and 636. He's gained weight, has enormous energy, his nose has cleared up. The **Mother Earth Cough Syrup** I just received but I don't think I will need it now because he is no longer coughing

Cayce's treatments seem so simple; it is hard to see how they could possibly work, when everything our doctors did so obviously failed.

Inspirol

"The inhalant seems to be doing the trick because my wife no longer has an asthma attack every time the weather changes."

From Washington

"The inhalant for colds and sinus is amazing – eases breathing, relieves a sinus headache. I have shared it with a number of friends who have been delighted, even with severe hay fever."

From Illinois

INDEX

BABY CARE

Supplementation:
- Lime water
- Herbal tea:
- Saffron tea
- Massage with:
- Cocoa butter
- Topical care:
- Alka-thyme
- Glycol-thymoline

BEAUTY/COMPLEXION

Supplementation:
- Formula 636/Formula 637
- Fragrance:
- Rosewater

Massage with:
- Aura Glow/Golden Magic
- Aura Glow Cream
- Dermaglow
- Sweet almond oil
- Gold Cream

BLOATING

Physical treatment:
- Spinal manipulation
- Colonics
- Massage

CALLUSES/CORNS

- Castor oil
- Casoda

CARBOHYDRATE INTOLERANCE

Supplementation:
- Ragweed tincture

CEREBROVASULAR HEALTH

Physical treatment:
- Electric vibrator
- Wet cell appliance
- Radiac (radio-active appliance)

CIRCULATORY SYSTEM HEALTH

Physical treatment:
- Massage
- Spinal manipulation
- Colonics

Supplementation:
- De-tense
- Atomidine
- Formula 545

Herbal tea:
- Watermelon seed tea
- Mullein tea leaves

Other treatment:
- Violet Ray

DIGESTIVE SUPPORT

Physical treatment:
- Spinal manipulation
- Massage

Supplementation:
- Formula 208
- Ragweed tincture
- Olive oil
- Limewater

Herbal tea:
- Elm bark tea
- American saffron tea

Hot/cold packs:
- Castor oil

DRY, UNCOMFORTABLE SKIN

Supplementation:
- Atomidine
- Sulflax

Herbal tea:
- Elm tea
- American saffron tea

Over-the-counter:
- Ray's liquid
- Ray's ointment

Topical care:
- Alka-thyme/Glycol- thymoline
- Camphor spirits
- Aura Glow/Golden Magic

ELIMINATION AIDS

Physical treatment:
- Wet cell appliance
- Radiac

Supplementation:
- Sulflax
- Olive oil
- Duogest

Herbal tea:
- American saffron tea

EYE CARE

Physical treatment:
- Spinal manipulation

Supplementation:
- Optikade
- Cola syrup

Herbal Tea:
- Watermelon seed tea

Hot/cold packs:
- Alka-thyme/Glyco-thymoline

FOOT CARE

Physical treatment:
- Massage
- Spinal manipulation

Massage with:
- Campho-derm
- Muscle treat

Topical care:
- Pedicure
- Sole Soother

HAIR CARE

Physical treatment:
- Spinal manipulation
- Massage
- Electric vibrator

Supplementation:
- Formula 545
- Atomidine
- Formula 636/Formula 637

Other treatments:
- Violet Ray

Topical care:
- Crudeoleum
- Crudeoleum rinse
- Pine tar shampoo
- Olive oil shampoo and conditioner
- Crudeoleum shampoo and conditioner
- Pine tar soap

HEMORRHOIDS

Physical treatment:
- Tim ointment

INSECT BITES

Physical treatment:
- Raise liquid
- Ray's ointment

JOINT CARE

Hot/cold packs
- Castor oil

Massage with:
- Peanut oil
- Egyptian oil
- Aura Glow
- Golden Magic

Other treatments:
- Hydrotherapy

LIVER HEALTH

Physical treatment:
- Spinal manipulation
- Massage
- Colonics

Supplementation:
- Olive oil
- Ragweed tincture
- Castor oil pack

MENOPAUSE

Supplementation:
- Atomidine
- Calcios
- Formula 636 /Formula 637

Other treatments:
- Violet Ray

MENSTRUATION

Supplementation:
- Formula 636/Formula 637

Other treatments:
- Violet Ray

MOLES

Physical treatment:
- Castor oil
- Casoda

MUSCLE TENSION

Physical treatment:
- Spinal manipulation
- Castor oil pack

Massage with:
- Muscle treat
- Campo-Derm
- Olive oil
- Egyptian oil
- Peanut oil
- Aura Glow
- Golden Magic

NERVOUS SYSTEM

Physical treatment:
- Spinal manipulation
- Massage
- Colonics

Supplementation:
- Sulflax
- Atomidine
- Formula 545

Herbal tea:
- Watermelon seed tea

Hot/cold packs:
- Alka-thyme
- Glyco-thymoline

Massage with:
- Olive oil
- Myrrh tincture
- Peanut oil
- Aura Glow
- Golden Magic
- Egyptian oil

Other treatments:
- Radiac
- Violet Ray
- Wet cell appliance

ORAL CARE

Supplementation:
- Atomidine
- Mouthwash/gargle:
- Glyco-thymoline
- Alka-thyme

Topical care:
- Ipsab
- Ipsab tooth powder

SUNBURN, MINOR BURNS AND SCRAPES

- Ray's liquid
- Ray's ointment

RELAXATION/TENSION RELIEF

Physical treatment:
- Electric vibrator

Supplementation:
- Valerian tincture
- Passionflower fusion

Physical treatment:
- Lithia water
- De-tense
- Castor oil pack

Massage with:
- Temple healer
- Olive oil

Other treatment:
- Radiac

RESPIRATORY SUPPORT

Inhalants:
- Inspirol
- Charred Oak Keg

Physical treatment:
- Spinal manipulation
- Massage

Supplementation:
- Atomidine
- Mothers Earth
- Ragweed tincture
- Calcious

Other treatments:
- Electric vibrator
- Carbon steel coin

Recommended Reading

1. The Oil that Heals by William A. McGarey

2. In Search of Healing by William A. McGarey

3. An Edgar Cayce Home Medicine Guide by Anonymous

If you enjoyed this book, would you be so kind as to leave a review on Amazon for others.

Go to EdgarCayceCures.com for more recommended reading and to learn more about the Edgar Cayce recommended remedies, therapies and treatments.

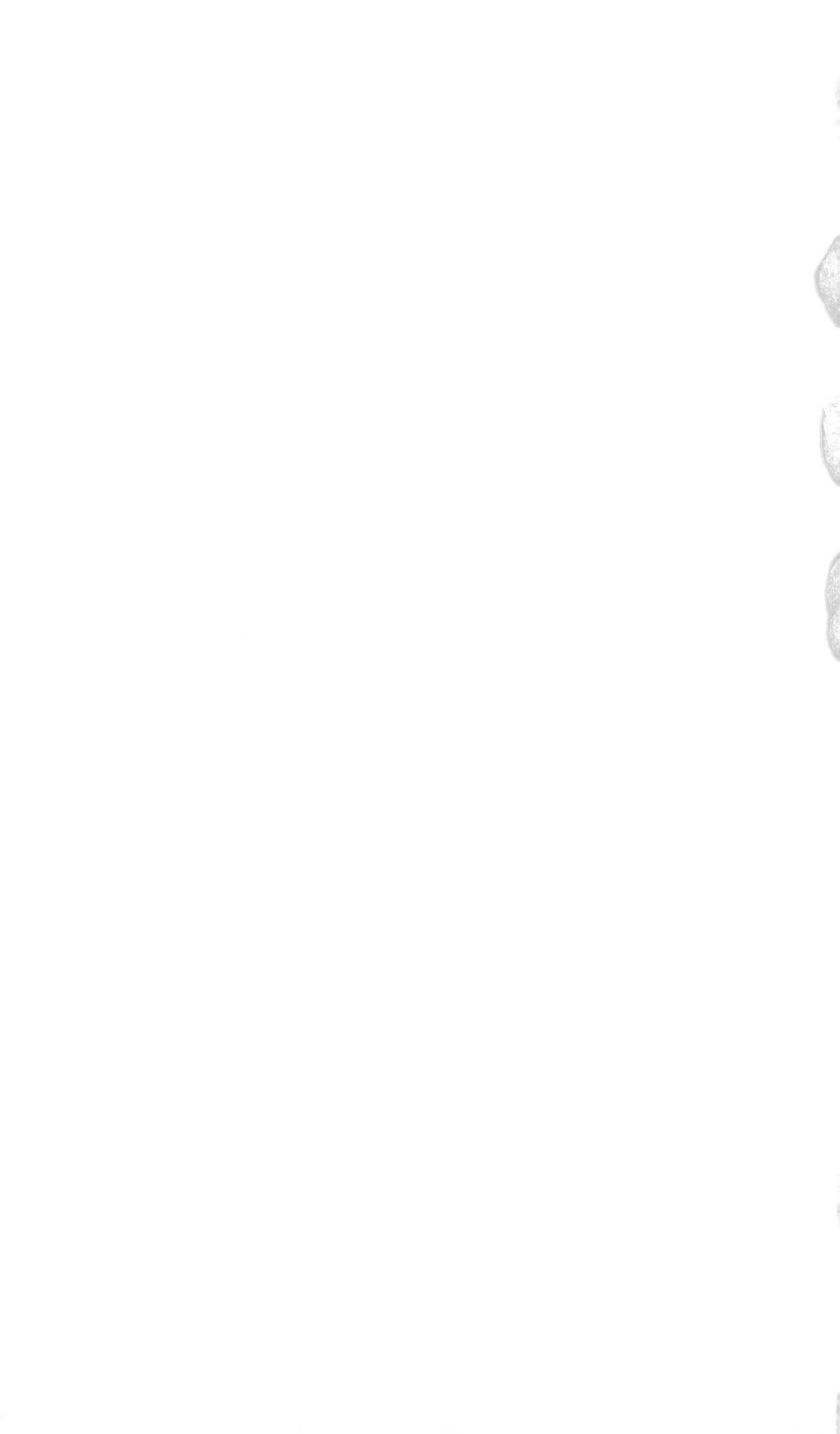

www.ingramcontent.com/pod-product-compliance
Lightning Source LLC
Chambersburg PA
CBHW061515180526
45171CB00001B/186